Ectomorpn
Diet

A Complete Guide on an
Ectomorphic Body Type

(Delicious Recipes to Improve Your Shape and Feel

Great Again)

Sharyl Davis

Published By **Andrew Zen**

Sharyl Davis

Ectomorph Diet: A Complete Guide on an Ectomorphic Body Type (Delicious Recipes to Improve Your Shape and Feel Great Again)

ISBN   978-1-77485-966-7

No part of this guidebook shall be reproduced in any form without permission in writing from the publisher except in the case of brief quotations embodied in critical articles or reviews.

Legal & Disclaimer

criminal intent, or under any other cause of action.

You agree to accept all risks of using the information presented inside this book. You need to consult a professional medical practitioner in order to ensure you are both able and healthy enough to participate in this program.

Table of contents

Chapter 1: What Is An Ectomorph?

The ectomorph is one of the three most common body types (somatotypes), characterized by a "thin frame" and difficulty to gain muscle mass as well as fat. People that belong to this somatotype are usually skinny, lean and have a high metabolic rate.

When exposed to a constant unhealthy diet and sedentary lifestyle, ectomorphs can actually gain some weight, which will most probably be belly fat, while their arms and legs will stay unusually thin.

Characteristics of the ectomorph body

Studies have shown that when strength training, the ectomorph body produces low levels of myogenin (a member of a large family of proteins

1

related by se𝟷uence homology, the helix-loop-helix (HLH) proteins. It is essential for the development of functional skeletal muscle.), which limits their capacity to build muscle mass.

In addition to the low muscle mass, the myogenin deficiency limits the energy reserves to the muscles and does not allow the ectomorph to train intensive and hard enough. This means that there is not enough stimulus for the muscles to grow. The Other Body Types

Along with an ectomorph, the other two body types (also referred to as somatotypes) include mesomorph (someone who typically has a sporty, athletic, or muscular build) and endomorph (a larger boned person who is curvier or has more fat on their body).

The good part about being an ectomorph

As mentioned before, ectomorphs have a really hard time putting some meat on their frame. This opens an opportunity for the ectomorph to eat more liberally, including junk food. Because of the fast metabolism, mos of the weight they put on them will be lean muscle rather than fat.

A fit and shredded body is an easy goal for the ectomorph; The effort they need to put in to create a visible six pack is really small. Most of the professional models belong to this somatotype.

 Training errors that ectomorphs make

– Too much cardio – if you are an ecto, you need to forget about long cardio sessions – ectomorphs are already skinny and lean enough, that too much cardio will only make things worse.

– Too many weight lifting sessions. Two to three weight lifting sessions a week are just enough for an ecto to make some progress. A bit more than this, and they will start losing weight again, by not allowing the muscles to recuperate.

Not sleeping enough How can ectomorphs gain muscle

Most of the training should revolve around the big basic moves: squats, bench press, shoulder press, deadlift, chin ups. Cut the isolation exercises as they do not provide enough stimulus for muscle growth.

Compound exercises performed with moderate to heavy weights and repetitions in the range of 5-8, will activate multiple joints and the larger muscle groups, which causes the body to produce testosterone and other anabolic hormones, important for gaining quality muscle. Which Popular Diets May Work Best for Ectomorphs

4

Lower-fat diets may feel like the stuff of the past, but they can work well for ectomorphs, including a vegan or vegetarian diet (that's filled with plenty of plant-based proteins). One diet that Catudal recommends against is the very high fat and low-carb ketogenic (keto) diet, "Particularly if your goal is to lose belly fat, a keto diet may increase [physical] stress, which will just prompt your body to hold onto excess weight," he says.

Food List for an Ectomorph

Ectomorphs tend to respond well to carbohydrates, so you can eat those freely. You'll just want to choose healthy sources, including fiber-rich fruits, veggies, and whole grains. To optimize your health, reach for plenty of protein, including from lean animal sources and plants like nuts and seeds. Prioritizing protein (along with strength training) will help with your muscle-building efforts.

Here are some of the foods you can eat on the ectomorph diet:

Meat and Fish

Chicken

Turkey

White fish (cod, mah-mahi)

Seafood (shrimp, scallops)

Eggs

Lean steak or beef

Dairy

Fat-free or low-fat yogurt or milk (keep to 1 serving a day)

Fruits and Vegetables

Berries

Mango

Oranges

Apples

Pears

Banana

Cauliflower

Green beans

Broccoli

Asparagus

Brussels sprouts

Squash

Nuts and Seeds

Almonds

Pistachios

Peanuts

Sunflower seeds

Pumpkin seeds

Grains and Starchy Vegetables

Whole-wheat bread

Old-fashioned or steel-cut oats

Brown rice

Quinoa

Farro

Sweet potato

Diet and Metabolism

Ectomorphs have a fast metabolism, which is both a blessing and a curse. A high metabolism makes is easy to get lean, and it can seem as if they can eat whatever they want and not gain weight. However, with age, their metabolisms will slow down, primarily due to low muscle mass, which can result in an unhealthy gain in body fat.

The best diet for an ectomorph is one that is higher in carbohydrates and calories. Approximately 50 to 60 percent of calories should come from carbs, 25 percent from protein and 25 percent from fat.

Additional Nutrition Tips

Eat every two to four hours.

Add at least 500 calories if you want to gain weight or muscle.

Choose warm foods over cold foods (better for digestion).

Best starchy carbohydrates include oats, brown rice, quinoa, sweet potatoes and potatoes.

Best fruit choices include bananas, mangoes, pineapple, papaya, avocado and peaches.

Best vegetable choices include broccoli, cauliflower, brussel sprouts, beets and carrots, especially cooked in coconut oil or ghee (clarified butter).

Nutrient dense snacks include nuts and seeds, as well as nut butters.

The key is to still eat a healthy, balanced diet rich in nutrients. Just because you have an ectomorph body type, doesn't mean you should use that as an excuse to eat everything, including junk food.

Pre- and Post-workout Nutrition

About 30 to 60 minutes before a workout, make sure to eat or drink a fast-digesting carbohydrate and some protein, such as fruit or toast with almond butter and jam. These nutrients will help keep you energized throughout your workout. And don't forget to stay hydrated before and during your workout. If your exercise lasts less than 60 minutes, hydrate with water. If it's longer than 60 minutes, consider adding a fast-digesting carb (gel, blocks, or beverage) to keep your energy level up.

Your post-workout meal should be consumed 30 to 60 minutes after your workout. The ideal post-workout meal includes a 3:1 or 4:1 ratio of carbs to protein to help quickly replenish your glycogen stores and repair and build muscle fibers.

Nutty And Fruity Amaranth Hot Cereal

(Makes 1 serving)

Ingredients

1/3 cup amaranth

2/3 cup water

1/4 cup rice milk

1/4 cup dried cranberries

1 Tbsp. chopped nuts

1 Tbsp. chia seeds

Directions

Bring water to a boil in a pot and add the amaranth. Cover and reduce heat to a simmer and cook until the water is absorbed. Stir in the rice milk, cranberries, nuts and chia seeds. Pour into a bowl and serve.

Fitness Goals

Ectomorphs are at a disadvantage when it comes to building muscle and sculpting the body. The goal of toning, sculpting and creating curves on a small, thin frame can be achieved with a dedicated training and nutrition program. All ectomorphs, whether his or her goal is to be a body builder or achieve a healthy, lean and strong body, can benefit from a solid, consistent weight-training program. Cardio

Ectomorphs tend to excel in endurance-type activities, so it's not surprising that many prefer cardio training over weight lifting. The key to stimulate muscle growth is to do the minimal amount of cardio required for general health. Three times a week for 30 minutes is recommended.

Weight Training

To build muscle mass, increase strength and sculpt the body, a simple weight-training routine using heavy weights is critical for the ectomorph. The focus should be on using heavier weights and completing three to five sets of approximately eight to 12 reps for each muscle group.

Weight Training Weekly Workout for Ectomorph:

Heavy weight, pyramid rep scheme

Day 1 – Chest/Triceps

Incline dumbbell press, 12, 10, 10, 8

Dumbbell flyes flat bench 3 x 12

Overhead extensions 12, 10, 10, 8

Dips 3 x 12

Day 2 – Back/Biceps

Wide-grip pull-ups 12, 10, 10, 8

Bent-over dumbbell rows 12, 10, 10, 8

Seated barbell curls 12, 10, 10, 8

Alternate dumbbell curls 3 x 12

Day 3 – Legs/Shoulders

Leg press 12, 10, 10, 8

Lying leg curls 12, 10, 10, 8

Barbell squats 3 x 12

Deadlifts 3 x 12

Walking lunges 3 x 12 each leg (total 24)

Military press 12, 10, 10, 8

Rear delt flyes 3 x 12

Lateral raise 3 x 12

Day 4 Rest/Slow Steady-state Cardio

Day 5 – Total-body Superset

Push-ups 3 x 12 with close grip lat. pulldown 3 x 12

Skull crushers 3 x 12 with standing biceps curls 3 x 12

Arnolds (shoulder press) 3 x 12 with step-ups 3 x 12 each leg

Days 6 and 7 Rest/Slow Steady-state Cardio

7 Beneficial Weight Gain Tips – Must Know Ectomorph Diet Rules

Tired of being called the 'skinny guy'? Always feel like you're the weakest in the gym? Being an ectomorph, for many, is just as bad as being an endomorph who's overweight.

 Try as you might, you just can't seem to put on weight – fat or muscle – and frustration sets in on a continual basis.

An ectomorph is described as someone who is naturally ⬚uite thin and has a metabolism that runs along at a rapid pace. Unfortunately, when you eat more, it just runs faster.

If you have this particular body type, you need to approach weight gain and muscle building differently than the average individual. Since your body doesn't act in an 'average' way, you can't use the same approach.

Let's look at seven ectomorph-specific weight gain tips that you need to know and abide by.

Tip #1: Do Less In The Gym

Contrary to what you might think, you should actually do less in the gym if you hope to gain weight. Far too many naturally thin people think that they need to be in the gym six days a week for at least an hour a day.

After all, since they are so thin, this must mean they need to do more to build muscle, right?

Wrong. The problem with this thinking is that it fails to realise that, as a skinny person, you just don't have the same recovery system that the average person does. Remember, muscle is built when you are resting. In the gym, you are actually breaking your muscle tissue down.

So the more time you spend in the gym and the less time you spend resting, the less time you are giving yourself to build that muscle mass.

An ectomorph should limit his gym sessions to 3-4 per week, staying in the gym for 45 minutes or so per session. That's all that's needed to see optimal results.

As you plan these sessions, be sure to focus more on compound movements and exercises, and less on the isolation work that you might be doing right now. You will get more of a hormonal response from the larger compound moves like squats, deadlifts, shoulder press, bench press and rows, which will in turn help you build muscle faster.

If you're too busy doing bicep curls, lateral raises, and leg extensions in the gym to focus on those above mentioned moves, your program is far less effective than it could be.

Tip #2: Track Those Calories

As an ectomorph, you might be putting yourself on a 'see-food' diet. Basically, if you see it, you eat it. In other words, you don't worry about tracking calories. Tracking calories is for those looking for weight loss, you may think.

Wrong. It's just as important for you to track calories as it is for someone who hopes to lose weight. Why? If you don't track calories, you have no way of knowing for sure how many you are getting in.

Most naturally thin people tend to overestimate the number of calories they're consuming,

22

meaning they're not eating nearly as much as they think they are. In order to see results, an ectomorph needs learn how to increase their calorie intake. If they aren't seeing results, it usually comes down to one simple reason: they aren't eating more calories than they are using.

Tracking calories is a simple and effective way of ensuring you are eating enough calories to see results. Tip #3: Prioritise Sleep

Prioritise Sleep

The next tip is to prioritise sleep. If you try and get by with six or seven hours of sleep, this could seriously be hindering your success.

Sleep is when your body goes into deep recovery mode and when you can be sure that you are recovering and building muscle. Sleep is also when your body releases growth hormones, which is a key to jumpstarting the rate that you are burning fat.

Aim for eight to nine hours of sleep a night. If building muscle is important to you, you need to find a way to incorporate this into your routine.

Tip #4: Ditch Food With A Low Calorie Density

As an ectomorph, you will want to avoid foods with a low calorie density.

What do we mean by that? Basically, avoid food that you need to eat a lot of in order to make any significant calorie gains.

A great example of food with a high calorie density is cooked oatmeal. A small serving will give you a big boost of energy and keep you feeling fuller for longer. A quarter cup of oatmeal will contain approximately 80 calories. Since your stomach can only hold so much food, so you will want to focus on getting the best 'bang for your buck', so to speak.

Some great calorie-dense foods include:

Nuts and nut butter

Whey protein powder

Bagels

Dried fruit

Avocados

Salmon

Grass-fed beef

Tip #5: Eat Every Few Hours

Eating little and often is a great way to ensure your body constantly has the fuel it requires.

If you have to eat 4000+ calories per day (which is not uncommon for most ectomorphs), it's far easier to get these calories in by dividing them up into 6-8 meals over the course of the day compared to 3 large, 1000+ calorie meals.

Your stomach simply won't handle that much food that well and you'll be left feeling sluggish for much of the day.

By fueling your body on a continuous basis and eating 400-500 calories per meal, you will keep your energy levels at a consistent level.

Make sure that each meal you eat contains a good levels of lean protein, complex carbohydrates and healthy fats to make it as balanced as possible.

Tip #6: Make Good Use Of Shakes

Another great way to get your calorie intake up is to make good use of shakes. These are convenient and quick options that will help you hit your daily calorie target. Blending together ingredients means you can up the calorie intake per serving.

Try adding in more calorie dense items into a 'weight gain' shake, such as nut butter, coconut oil, flaxseeds, avocado, cottage cheese, Greek yogurt, or ground up oatmeal.

Do steer clear of commercially prepared weight gainers however. While these may seem like a good idea, as many have 500+ calories per scoop, they are often loaded with sugar and are only going to provide your body with empty calories. They will leave you feeling hungry again quite quickly and won't give you the nutrition that you need.

Prepare your own so that you can control exactly what goes into each shake.

Tip #7: Watch Your Extra Activity

Finally, the last tip to remember is to watch your extra activity level. Those who are ectomorphs tend to be rather fidgety in nature, meaning try as they might, they just can't sit still.

They may find that they tend to pace around often, jiggle their foot, or are constantly doing other activities throughout the day because they are so restless.

If this is you, it's time to focus on slowing down.

All this extra activity is going to dramatically increase your total daily calorie burn, meaning you will need to eat even more food than you already do to gain weight.

All this extra activity is actually a prominent reason in explaining why many ectomorphs have that particular body type.

If you can relax and slow down a bit, you might come to find that you will achieve your weight gain goals a little easier.

This will take you some time to get rid of this habit as it's something that's been ingrained in you. But, if you can look at your overall daily schedule and try and find ways to relax and take it easy more often, you'll soon get used to it.

So there you have some of the best tips for any ectomorph who is trying to build muscle to know and remember. It's vital that you make some adjustments to how you are living, exercising and eating or you will not see the desired results.

Chapter 2: A 7-Day Sample Menu For The Ectomorph Body Type

Day 1

Breakfast Old-fashioned or steel-cut oatmeal topped with strawberries and walnuts

Snack Hard-boiled egg and soy milk latte

Lunch Mediterranean quinoa salad with chopped veggies and olive oil

Snack Apple and almonds

Dinner Turkey and mango tacos wrapped in lettuce leaves served with a side of black beans

Day 2

Breakfast Smoothie made with fruit, almond milk, and protein powder

Snack Trail mix made with nuts and dried fruit

Lunch Avocado toast topped with a fried egg, side salad

Snack Carrots and black bean dip

Dinner Sliced flank steak fajitas with onions and peppers wrapped in sprouted whole-grain tortillas

Day 3

Breakfast Sweet potato toast topped with a thin smear of nut butter and turkey bacon

Snack Pear with mixed nuts

Lunch Bean and veggie burger served on a whole-grain bun, side of steamed broccoli

Snack Protein bar

Dinner Grilled chicken, sautéed kale, tomato and cucumber salad, side of farro

Day 4

Breakfast Whole-grain toast with fat-free or low-fat Greek yogurt and a sliced pear

Snack Protein bar

Lunch Mixed greens salad with chopped vegetables, roasted turkey, and vinaigrette

Snack Apple and a slice of cheese

Dinner Chicken and mushroom stir-fry over brown rice

Day 5

Breakfast Slice of veggie frittata with roasted sweet potatoes

Snack Banana with almond butter

Lunch Tuna mashed with avocado on whole grain crackers, side salad

Snack Protein bar

Dinner Quinoa bake made with tomato sauce, mixed vegetables, and chicken

Day 6

Breakfast Fat-free or low-free Greek yogurt parfait with chopped apples, walnuts, whole-grain cereal, and cinnamon

Snack Small smoothie with protein powder

Lunch Turkey chili and a side salad with vinaigrette

Snack Sliced veggies dipped in homemade guacamole

Dinner Grilled shrimp and vegetables kabobs on a bed of quinoa

Day 7

Breakfast Overnight oats made with fat-free or low-fat yogurt, almond milk, and topped with raspberries

Snack Hard-boiled egg, piece of fruit

Lunch Turkey sandwich on whole-grain bread, mashed avocado, lettuce, tomato, onion, baby carrots on the side

Snack Broccoli dipped in hummus

Dinner Roasted cod, Brussels sprouts, baked sweet potato

Advantages of the Ectomorph Diet

Compared to the eating plans for mesomorphs and endomorphs, the ectomorph diet is higher in carbs. So if you're averse to low-carb diets, you may find this eating plan meshes well with your tastes — and that's great, so long as you eat carbs in moderation. Yet as the ectomorph diet advises, by increasing the amount of protein you eat per day and combining it with weight training recommendations (below), you'll stimulate your body to build more muscle.

The benefit of this is that not only does an increase in muscle mass boost your metabolism, as Harvard Health Publishing notes, but it can also protect your bones as you age. As research published in April 2019 in the International Journal of Environmental Research and Public Health noted, losing muscle mass was linked to 2.5-fold greater odds of osteoporosis.

Disadvantages of the Ectomorph Diet

You'll need to make sure you're eating enough protein (100 to 150 grams per day) in order to build muscle and tone up, says Catudal. And, it may feel counterintuitive to snack on tuna or hardboiled eggs in the afternoon if your go-to before was crackers or an apple.

That said, if you're a hybrid ectomorph and are carrying excess fat around your waist, Melina Jampolis, MD, an internist and board-certified physician nutrition specialist in Valley Village, California, would not recommend a higher carb diet for you. "Many patients who have been thin their whole lives gain weight in their belly," she says. In that case, limiting high-starch choices like pasta and bread in favor of sweet potatoes, oats, and beans may be advised, according to the thinking behind the body type diet. "The good news," she suggests, "is that this body tends to respond very quickly to cutting carbs and they can lose weight efficiently," she says.

Still, keep in mind that there's no one perfect diet for everyone. And if weight loss is what you're after, another diet plan, such as one that limits calories instead of carbs, can help you reach your goal, as a study published in July 2019 in The Lancet noted.

Furthermore, the body type diet does not have rigorous scientific research supporting its use; therefore, there's no proof it will result in weight loss or any health benefits.

Ectomorph Diet

Ectomorphs don't have to count the calories. They can usually eat pretty liberally and eat as much as possible. This, however, doesn't mean that ectos can turn exclusively to junk food or overeat on sweets. Remember to stick to a healthy diet, containing protein from lean meats, low fat dairy, eggs and fish as well as complex carbs.

The amount of protein consumed per day should be in the range of 1 – 1.5 grams per LB of body weight. The amount of carbs should be anywhere around 2 grams per LB up to 4 grams per LB of body weight.

Muscle building supplements

1. Protein shakes – they are essential of you want to get all your protein on a daily basis, but you are

not able to eat enough foods. You can combine whey, egg and casein throughout the day. The post-workout shake should be whey because of the faster absorption, the shake before sleep can be either egg or casein.

2. Take BCAA before exercise, they will provide the body with more energy and sustain anabolic process.

3. Add 10 grams of creatine a day, which not only increases the volume of the muscle cells, but also improves energy processes.

To sum it up : The basic rules on training/nutrition for ectomorphs

– short but intense training up to three times a week,

– focus on the basic exercises,

– eat at least 1 gram of protein and 2 grams of carbs per LB of body weight per day.

Nutrition Tip

Ectomorphs looking to gain weight and muscle mass should follow these basic tips:

Quality Calories —Remember that you are what you eat; junk in = junk out. If you wish to gain weight as an ectomorph, consume a lot of quality calories to obtain true growth.

Eat Often – Your body burns through food quickly so you need a constant stream of nutrients being delivered to help rebuild your muscles following your training.

Eat Before Bed – A high-quality protein source before bed helps ensure your body has the building blocks it needs during the time it does the most repairs (while you're asleep).

A Solid Meal Composition – Build your meals to fit your specific needs. An Ectomorph should try to include 1-2 palms of protein, 1-2 fists of veggies, 2-3 handfuls of carb-dense food, and a source of healthy fats in your major meals.

Nutrition Rules for Every Ectomorph

Take Advantage of Carbs

A much higher percentage of your caloric intake should come from carbohydrates. The nice thing about carbs is that we can eat boat-loads of them without getting full. Use that to your advantage by eating a generous serving of carbs at every meal. Starchy, unprocessed, whole grain carbs will help you feel and look your best—opt for sweet potatoes over white bread. Drink simple carbs during your workout. If anyone should be drinking calories, it's the ectomorph. You'll feel energized and have more to give, especially towards the end of a grueling workout. Don't get in the habit of drinking sugary carbs all day, however. Outside of your workout window (from the start of your workout until about an hour after your last lift), keep your carbs unprocessed, starchy, and whole, as mentioned above.

Don't Skimp on Protein

Also have a post workout protein shake. That's right, in addition to a carb drink during the workout, you should have a protein shake immediately after your workout. Post workout protein does wonders for recovery and allows your hard work in the gym to pay off. Adding some carbs to your shake (berries, honey, almond milk) is a way to sneak in some extra calories and make your shake delightfully delicious. Push your calorie intake until you start gaining mass. You want to do the exact opposite of someone trying to lose weight. Add about 500 calories to your diet and see if your weight starts to increase. If it doesn't, try reducing your non-resistance exercise (any cardio-based exercise). Still no weight-gain? Add another 500 calories to your diet. Repeat until the scale starts to move.

Pace Yourself

You need to eat every two to four hours. Because your metabolic rate is so fast, you need to constantly be fueling your engine. If you want to get bigger, eating needs to become your job. Endomorphs (naturally broad and "thick-boned") also need to eat often but for exactly the opposite reasons. For endomorphs it helps with control, for ectomorphs it helps with excess.

All About Balance

Protein requirements are still important. Like all good eaters, you should be eating protein with every meal. That means eggs for breakfast, mid-morning nuts (which are mostly fat, but contain protein), chicken for lunch, a post workout protein shake, and steak for dinner. Mmm. Manhood. Fruits and vegetables are still important. Vitamins, minerals and phytonutrients are in these foods that are absolutely essential for you to grow and be healthy. Don't allow ectomorphia to be an excuse to eat crap. A healthy diet always includes plants also with every meal. Ultimately, getting bigger is not an easy task for the ectomorph. Most of the information out there is about weight loss. Some of those rules need to be broken and some of those rules still apply. But a smart nutrition plan will make all of the difference when going from she-man to He-Man.

How Protein Before Bed Can Promote Muscle Growth

Whether you want to lose weight or gain it, a diet with an adeᵒuate amount of protein is key.

The Dietary Guidelines for Americans suggest your daily calories should consist of:

10 to 35 percent of protein

45 to 65 percent from carbohydrates

20 to 35 percent of fat

The recommended daily allowance of protein is 0.8 grams per kilogram of body weight. Research suggests, though, that athletes benefit from more protein to maximize muscle growth. Those who frequently and consistently lift weights or do resistance training may benefit from consuming 1.3 to 1.8 grams of protein per kilogram of body weight per day.

That means that an active 180-pound male should consume about 106 to 147 grams of protein a day for muscle growth. An active 140-pound woman should consume between 83 and 114 grams of protein per day.

Is there an optimal time to consume this protein? While hitting the overall daily intake is most important, research does suggest that protein timing can make a difference.

Studies are mixed about whether consuming protein immediately after a workout has a beneficial effect on muscle growth. Several studies do show that protein consumed before bed can indeed foster muscle growth.

The science behind it

Protein supplies amino acids, which build our muscles. Our muscles repair themselves and grow while we sleep. Growth hormone is elevated during this time. This hormone boosts muscle growth and decreases fat.

Studies have shown that if you consume an ample amount of protein right before bed, you'll take full advantage of this spike in growth hormone and maximize muscle gains. This happens because you're providing the amino acids that are needed for repair and growth.

A 2012 study assessed the effect of eating protein before bed with 16 healthy young male participants. They performed a single bout of weightlifting in the evening and were provided 20 grams of protein immediately after exercise. Thirty minutes before sleep, eight of the men ingested a beverage with 40 grams of casein. Muscle protein synthesis rates were increased in the eight men who consumed the casein beverage before bed. This provided evidence that protein increases postexercise overnight recovery.

Another study from 2015 monitored 44 young men as they completed a 12-week resistance training program. All participants consumed a high-protein diet (1.3 grams of protein per kilogram of body weight). One group consumed a drink before bed containing 27.5 grams of protein and 15 grams of carbohydrates. The other group received a placebo drink. The group who consumed the protein drink saw greater improvements in muscle strength, muscle size, and muscle fiber size.

However, both of these studies had limitations. It's not clear in both studies whether the increase in total daily protein intake or the protein intake specifically before bed resulted in muscle gains.

However, the overall body of research on protein intake and muscle growth has led the International Society of Sports Nutrition to take the stance that "casein protein (~ 30-40 g) prior to sleep can acutely increase MPS [muscle protein synthesis] and metabolic rate throughout the night." They recommend nighttime protein intake for athletes who train in the early morning without eating, or in the evening after dinner.

And in a different 2015 study comparing carbohydrate snacks verses protein snacks before sleep, the protein group had improved metabolism.

Supplements vs. real food

While protein powders, shakes, and bars may also provide an adequate amount of protein, it's preferable to consume "real" food instead at most meals.

These supplements don't offer the same nutrients as whole foods like lean meats, eggs, or yogurt. They're also often packed with sugar or artificial sweeteners and may be high in calories. What's more, supplements aren't strictly regulated by the U.S. Food and Drug Administration. That said, the studies mentioned above did use protein supplements, not mixed protein meals.

If you have trouble meeting your daily recommended caloric or protein needs, a protein shake could be a good option. The U.S. Department of Agriculture recommends about

2,600 calories a day for a moderately active man and 2,000 calories a day for a moderately active woman for weight maintenance. If you're aiming to lose weight, your calorie needs will be lower.

What Is Ectomorph Body Type?

An ectomorph body type refers to the type of body with lean muscles & weak-looks. For example, a girl with an ectomorph body type has narrow shoulders and long limbs. Girls with this body type often find it challenging to gain muscles and weight. The main reason behind this is their super-quick metabolism rate. Thus, everything they eat during the whole day gets burnt very quickly. This is why ectomorph girls are not able to put on weight easily and need a special diet for it. Therefore, we have prepared the best safe weight gain diet for people with an ectomorph body type.

Why Bother Knowing Your Body Type?

Not every body type is created equal and there are hundreds of factors that can influence our ability to achieve our fitness goals. At its core, our ability to achieve our fitness goals are largely influenced by 3 main things: our genetics, diet, and exercise plan.

Our genetics are responsible for the development of our body type and unfortunately, we have no say in this matter. Like the cards you are dealt during a poker game, our genetics is something that we cannot control. Some people are dealt aces and others are dealt seven deuce. Regardless of the cards you've been dealt, you can still achieve any fitness goal you set your mind to. They key is patience, persistence, and to focus on what you can control. Which brings me to my next point.

The two things you can control are your diet and exercise plan. Think of each component as wild cards, in which you can play either card, in any scenario, to your advantage.

How The Body Type Diet Works And How To

Know If You're An Ectomorph

You may also categorize yourself as an ectomorph if you know you don't gain weight easily. "These are the tall, thin people in the gym, and they're often male. They're trying to put on muscle and get stronger," says Nanci Guest, PhD, RD, a nutritional scientist and personal trainer in Toronto. Yet she's quick to point out that it's usually not a matter of your specific body type, but rather, it's probably genetics. "We have genes that determine if you have a faster or slower metabolism," she says. And it's these metabolism-revving genes that are mostly responsible for a thin body frame.

You might also find that you can (or could) "eat whatever you want" and not gain weight —

something that sounds ideal in theory, but an unhealthy diet can have an effect on your health no matter what your weight or body mass index (BMI).

Ectomorph Hybrid Types

Over time, says Catudal, ectomorphs can become one of the common hybrid types, an "ecto-endomorph," characterized by long limbs but a bigger belly from a sedentary lifestyle and less than stellar eating habits.

As you age, that state of "skinny fat" — a term for people who are normal weight but have excess fat mass — can catch up to your long-term health, per the Mayo Clinic. A study published in January 2018 in Clinical Interventions in Aging found that having low lean body mass (muscle) and excess fat was associated with a greater risk of developing cognitive problems.

Which Popular Diets May Work Best For

Ectomorphs

Lower-fat diets may feel like the stuff of the past, but they can work well for ectomorphs, including a vegan or vegetarian diet (that's filled with plenty of plant-based proteins). One diet that Catudal recommends against is the very high fat and low-carb ketogenic (keto) diet, "Particularly if your goal is to lose belly fat, a keto diet may increase [physical] stress, which will just prompt your body to hold onto excess weight," he says.

Ectomorph Diet Plan Principles

Now that you know who are ectomorphs and whether or not you fall into this category, let's

move ahead to next section on this article —
Ectomorph diet plan principles.

Eat Surplus Calories

It goes without saying that for ectomorphs to gain
muscle and put on weight, they will have to start
eating more calories than they usually do. Unlike
the popular belief, tracking calories is as
important for ectomorphs as those on a weight-
loss diet. So, how will you do it?

To begin with, calculate the total number of
calories you consume each day. You can use
Myfitnesspal Calorie Chart for the same. Once
you know your gross calorie intake, it's time to
calculate your daily calorie expenditure by using
Calorie Calculator. If values of both intake calories
and expenditure are e?ual, then you are going to
see almost no gains.

The trick is to increase the intake calories by atleast 250-350 each day so that by the end of the week you are likely to have put on atleast half a pound of weight.

Eat High Calorie Dense Food

Taking a cue from the first principle, an ectomorph needs to eat enough food all day long. Having said that, it's also important for ectomorphs to consider the calorie density of the food they are eating. Alright, let me make it easy for you.

Being an ectomorph, you may want to skip all the food items with low calorie density aka food items you need to consume in huge quantity to make considerable calorie gains. For instance, a small bowl of cooked oatmeal contains just about

100-120 calories but proves very effective in suppressing your hunger and making you feel full.

Hence, ectomorphs are suggested to avoid such foods and choose high calorie-dense foods like dried fruits, meat, fish and whey protein.

Eat Frequently

Well, if truth be told, eating three meals a day won't work at all. Once you are on an ectomorph diet, you will have to eat atleast 6-8 meals each day and that too at freﬗuent intervals. Out of these meals, have at least 3 major meals and 3 small meals or snacks.

I would advise to keep breakfast, lunch, and dinner as main meals and adding healthy snacks to the routine between each of these meals. This way, not only you will able to keep energy levels high throughout the day but also ease the process of weight gain which may be a difficult task to accomplish otherwise.

Use Protein Shakes

Who said protein shakes are just for elite athletes and bodybuilders? An average skinny gym goer can also use protein shakes for his benefit in many ways. First and foremost, protein shakes especially the ones made with high-quality whey isolate are among the finest ways to increase the protein intake. On top of it, protein shakes can help ectomorphs to achieve their daily calorie target with ease. Along with whey protein, add ingredients like oats, peanut butter, fresh fruits, and yogurt to your protein shake.

Responding to a common query that I receive quite often regarding the use of mass gainers for weight gain for ectomorphs, I would advise you to avoid all sorts of gainers at all cost. Although weight gainers contain a lot of calories, they are fully loaded with sugars and artificial additives.

Relying completely upon weight gainers may prove to be fatal in the long run. Instead of using mass gainers, I would suggest you use a better source of complete protein like whey protein and casein protein.

What Can You Eat?

Here are some of the expert-recommended calorie-dense foods to help in boosting weight gain for ectomorphs.

Salmon – Salmon is one of the most nutritious and calorie-dense foods in the world. A small portion of salmon is filled with healthy fats and cálories, which are effective for boosting weight gain. Moreover, salmon is loaded with nutrition like minerals, vitamins, antioxidants, protein, and omega-3 fatty acids. All these elements help in promoting the overall body healthy by preventing many diseases. Thus, including it in your weight gain diet plan will speed up the process greatly.

Protein Powders – Apart from being a healthy source of protein, protein supplements are great for weight gain. Various milk-based protein powders like whey & casein can help in increasing your weight healthily. These are also filled with healthy calories to build your muscles faster. For best results, you can prepare protein drinks with the powder and drink it before or after a gym workout. Also, it is recommended to go for unflavored powder and trusted brands.

Avocado – Avocado is undoubtedly the most nutritious & calorie-dense fruit in the world. Moreover, these are also filled with healthy fats that help in boosting the weight gain process. Apart from this, avocados are rich in fiber, vitamins, minerals, folic acid, and omega-3 fatty acids. All these nutrients not only help you to put on weight healthily but also prevent several health issues also herbal remedies for weight gain. A large avocado can easily offer 300+ calories to you.

Nuts & nut butter – Nuts are a great source of healthy fats and good calories, which is why they're good for gaining weight. Apart from this, nuts are also filled with vitamins, minerals, dietary fiber, protein, and other essential nutrients. All these elements promote your overall health while providing you with much-needed calories. Moreover, you can always eat nuts in the form of nut butter, like a spread over bread. Also, avoid buying nut butter with artificial sweeteners & hydrogenated oils.

Red meat – Red meat is a great source of protein and healthy fats that help in accelerating your weight gain process. Furthermore, red meat is loaded with nutrients like vitamins, minerals, and omega-3 fatty acids. Because of this, red meat is considered to be great for overall health as well. Also, make sure to get leaner parts of the red meat to avoid heart-related problems. Some examples of red meat include pork, mutton, etc.

Starchy foods – Starchy foods are an excellent source of carbohydrates and healthy calories. Moreover, these foods are loaded with minerals, vitamins, healthy fats, dietary fiber, and phytonutrients. Also, several medical studies have linked the consumption of starchy foods with muscle & weight gain. Thus, you need to add foods rich in starch to your diet plan. Some examples of starch-rich foods include whole-grain bread, quinoa, whole-grain cereals

Dried fruits – Dried fruits are also having various nutrients and healthy calories to help boost weight loss. Moreover, these contain vitamins, minerals, protein, and antioxidants. This is why the consumption of dried fruits is links wiht improvement in overall health. Apart from this, several studies have shown positive weight gain effects of dried fruits due to high calorie-count. Some of the most calorie-dense dried fruits include apricot, date, fig, and raisins, etc.

Dark chocolate – Dark chocolate is another great food for weight gain, as it has healthy fats and calories. Furthermore, it is rich in zinc, iron, antioxidants, and magnesium. Thus, it is a very healthy option to put on some weight. Also, make sure to get dark chocolate with more than 70% cacao content for better heart health. Other health benefits of dark chocolate include healthier skin, better blood circulation, and cholesterol regulation.

Eggs – Eggs are one of the most nutritious and calorie-dense foods on the planet. Eggs are rich in vitamins, minerals, protein, antioxidants, selenium, and healthy fats. This is why eggs are considered to be great for boosting muscle growth and weight gain. Therefore, experts recommend girls with ectomorph body type to add eggs in their diet plan.

Milk – Milk is another nutrient dense food, which contains all sorts of healthy calories and nutrients for weight gain. Furthermore, milk is a great source of vitamins, minerals, healthy fats, carbohydrates, and protein. All these elements are effective in boosting muscle development and weight gain. Several medical studies have linked the consumption of skim milk with an increase in weight. Thus, you need to add milk to your daily diet plan for better results.

Rice – Rice is a great calorie-dense food having healthy carbohydrates and calories to boost weight gain. Moreover, rice is an excellent source of vitamins, minerals, dietary fiber, and energy. A large cup of rice can offer you 200+ calories easily. You can always combine it with other calorie-dense foods like legumes, to get better results in less time.

Homemade protein smoothies (HPS) – Homemade protein smoothies are a great option to put on weight in a healthy and nutritious way. The best thing about HPS is that you can easily prepare them according to your taste & nutrition requirements. You can add protein powder, fruits, nuts, and dried fruits, etc. to increase the total calorie count of the drink. Moreover, you can easily find several recipes of homemade protein smoothies on the internet.

Food List For An Ectomorph

Ectomorphs tend to respond well to carbohydrates, so you can eat those freely. You'll just want to choose healthy sources, including fiber-rich fruits, veggies, and whole grains. To optimize your health, reach for plenty of protein, including from lean animal sources and plants like nuts and seeds. Prioritizing protein (along with strength training) will help with your muscle-building efforts.

Here are some of the foods you can eat on the ectomorph diet:

Meat and Fish

• Chicken

• Turkey

• White fish (cod, mah-mahi)

• Seafood (shrimp, scallops)

• Eggs

• Lean steak or beef

Dairy

• Fat-free or low-fat yogurt or milk (keep to 1 serving a day)

Fruits and Vegetables

• Berries

- Mango

- Oranges

- Apples

- Pears

- Banana

- Cauliflower

- Green beans

- Broccoli

- Asparagus

- Brussels sprouts

- S?uash

Nuts and Seeds

- Almonds

• Pistachios

• Peanuts

• Sunflower seeds

• Pumpkin seeds

Grains and Starchy Vegetables

• Whole-wheat bread

• Old-fashioned or steel-cut oats

• Brown rice

• Quinoa

• Farro

• Sweet potato

Diet And Metabolism

Ectomorphs have a fast metabolism, which is both a blessing and a curse. A high metabolism makes is easy to get lean, and it can seem as if they can eat whatever they want and not gain weight. However, with age, their metabolisms will slow down, primarily due to low muscle mass, which can result in an unhealthy gain in body fat.

The best diet for an ectomorph is one that is higher in carbohydrates and calories. Approximately 50 to 60 percent of calories should come from carbs, 25 percent from protein and 25 percent from fat.

Additional Nutrition Tips

• Eat every two to four hours.

• Add at least 500 calories if you want to gain weight or muscle.

• Choose warm foods over cold foods (better for digestion).

• Best starchy carbohydrates include oats, brown rice, quinoa, sweet potatoes and potatoes.

• Best fruit choices include bananas, mangoes, pineapple, papaya, avocado and peaches.

• Best vegetable choices include broccoli, cauliflower, brussel sprouts, beets and carrots, especially cooked in coconut oil or ghee (clarified butter).

• Nutrient dense snacks include nuts and seeds, as well as nut butters.

The key is to still eat a healthy, balanced diet rich in nutrients. Just because you have an ectomorph body type, doesn't mean you should use that as an excuse to eat everything, including junk food.

Pre- And Post-Workout Nutrition

About 30 to 60 minutes before a workout, make sure to eat or drink a fast-digesting carbohydrate and some protein, such as fruit or toast with almond butter and jam. These nutrients will help keep you energized throughout your workout. And don't forget to stay hydrated before and during your workout. If your exercise lasts less than 60 minutes, hydrate with water. If it's longer than 60 minutes, consider adding a fast-digesting carb (gel, blocks, or beverage) to keep your energy level up.

Your post-workout meal should be consumed 30 to 60 minutes after your workout. The ideal post-workout meal includes a 3:1 or 4:1 ratio of carbs to protein to help quickly replenish your glycogen stores and repair and build muscle fibers. Here's an example of a great post-workout meal breakfast cookbook.

Nutty And Fruity Amaranth Hot Cereal

(Makes 1 serving)

• 1/3 cup amaranth

• 2/3 cup water

• 1/4 cup rice milk

• 1/4 cup dried cranberries

• 1 Tbsp. chopped nuts

• 1 Tbsp. chia seeds

1. Bring water to a boil in a pot and add the amaranth. Cover and reduce heat to a simmer and cook until the water is absorbed. Stir in the

rice milk, cranberries, nuts and chia seeds. Pour into a bowl and serve.

Fitness Goals

Ectomorphs are at a disadvantage when it comes to building muscle and sculpting the body. The goal of toning, sculpting and creating curves on a small, thin frame can be achieved with a dedicated training and nutrition program. All ectomorphs, whether his or her goal is to be a body builder or achieve a healthy, lean and strong body, can benefit from a solid, consistent weight-training program.

Weight Training

To build muscle mass, increase strength and sculpt the body, a simple weight-training routine using heavy weights is critical for the ectomorph. The focus should be on using heavier weights and completing three to five sets of approximately eight to 12 reps for each muscle group.

82

Weight Training Weekly Workout for Ectomorph:

Heavy weight, pyramid rep scheme

Day 1 – Chest/Triceps

Incline dumbbell press, 12, 10, 10, 8

Dumbbell flyes flat bench 3 x 12

Overhead extensions 12, 10, 10, 8

Dips 3 x 12

Day 2 – Back/Biceps

Wide-grip pull-ups 12, 10, 10, 8

Bent-over dumbbell rows 12, 10, 10, 8

Seated barbell curls 12, 10, 10, 8

Alternate dumbbell curls 3 x 12

Day 3 – Legs/Shoulders

Leg press 12, 10, 10, 8

Lying leg curls 12, 10, 10, 8

Barbell squats 3 x 12

Deadlifts 3 x 12

Walking lunges 3 x 12 each leg (total 24)

Military press 12, 10, 10, 8

Rear delt flyes 3 x 12

Lateral raise 3 x 12

Day 4 Rest/Slow Steady-state Cardio

Day 5 – Total-body Superset

Push-ups 3 x 12 with close grip lat. pulldown 3 x 12

Skull crushers 3 x 12 with standing biceps curls 3 x 12

Arnolds (shoulder press) 3 x 12 with step-ups 3 x 12 each leg

Days 6 and 7 Rest/Slow Steady-state Cardio

Which Exercises Are Best For Ectomorphs?

It is important to remember that not everyone you meet has the same fitness goals. Whether it is to gain muscle, lose fat, or maintain your physique, everyone has or should have their own definition of fitness success. That being said, recommending the best exercises for any particular individual will depend largely on their personal goals.

In my experience, ectomorphs, aka hardgainers, typically want one thing… to gain muscle mass! They are tired of spending countless hours in the gym, working harder and longer than their peers, only to see minimal gains. So what's the missing link?

First, you are probably not eating enough. If you understand the concept of energy balance, you'll realize that if you are not gaining weight while working out hard, you are not providing your muscles with the needed energy and nutrients to grow. So the first thing you should do is eat more.

Alright. You've started eating steak and eggs, potatoes and whatnot. The next tip I'll give you is this: Compound exercises.

What are examples of compound exercises?

I will say it again, compound exercises! Compound exercises build the most muscle mass and increase strength the fastest. And yes, this includes lean body mass for those who want to avoid putting on bulky muscle mass.

This is because compound movements hit numerous muscle groups as you perform multi-joint movements through a range of motion. From an effort standpoint, if you are an ectomorph and are neglecting these essential exercises, this is a recipe for maximum input with little output. So what are these compound exercises you speak of?

Glad you asked. There are a wide variety of fun and beneficial compound exercises to choose from. Below, I have narrowed down my top three favorite compound exercises that I incorporate into my routine every week:

1. Flat Bench Press

• Lie face up on a flat bench, with your back slightly arched, buttocks on the bench, and feet flat on the floor.

• Grab the barbell with an overhand grip, slightly wider than shoulder width apart.

• Inhale and lower the bar to chest level, until elbows are parallel to the ground.

• Maintain control of the bar, and extend the arms back up while exhaling to end the movement.

2. Squat

• Slide under the barbell and place it on the trapezius, slightly above the posterior deltoid. Grab the bar tightly with the hands, and look straight ahead.

• Inhale and contract the abdominal muscles to prevent the torso from collapsing forward, arch the back slightly, and remove the bar from the stand.

• Step back a few inches, place both feet slightly wider than shoulder width and point toes slightly outward.

• Bend forward from the hips, and continue the movement until the thighs are slightly below parallel to the ground.

• Straighten the legs and lift the torso to the starting position, then exhale.

3. Deadlift

• Stand facing the barbell, legs shoulder width apart, abdominals contracted, and back slightly arched.

- Bend the knees until the thighs are parallel to the ground, and grab the barbell using one overhand grip, and underhand grip.

- Inhale, lift the barbell by straightening the legs and then contract the back at the top portion of the movement.

- While keeping your back straight, proceed to lower the barbell releasing at the hips and bending your knees until your thighs are once again parallel to the ground or the weight touches the floor.

- Exhale at the end of the movement.

Pace Yourself!

An important concept to keep in mind during your training is that if you are an ectomorph, less is more. You don't need to work out harder or longer than your peers in order to keep up with them.

What your workouts should be is intense and shorter in length. Focus on big muscle groups and limit your workouts to 45-60 minutes max.

Lastly, exercise strategically and always beware of over training. Each compound exercise should be performed to reach muscle failure within the 4-8 rep range. That means, by the time you complete your eighth rep, you are incapable of completing a ninth rep due to muscle failure or fatigue.

That is a good thing! The tension being put on the muscle from the weight is optimal within that rep range. Whereas, if you notice yourself completing your eighth rep with enough strength to pump out a few more reps, that is a sign that you need to increase the weight. If the tension isn't intense enough it won't stimulate any muscle growth. Simple as that!

What About Cardio?

Cardiovascular activity has amazing benefits for heart health among a long list of other benefits. Among these benefits include an increased metabolic rate, which means an easier time maintaining your weight or losing weight as the case may be.

Wait, don't ectomorphs already have a more efficient metabolism?

My point exactly! Ectomorphs have a relatively more efficient metabolism and are at a disadvantage when it comes to adding size because of that. Therefore, proceed to engage in cardio, but do so sparingly. Stick to the simplest forms such as walking, jogging, or playing your favorite sport. Again, and I cannot stress this enough: you need to stay in a positive energy balance. And cardio will make it harder to do so.

It is always a great idea to perform cardio as a way to increase heart rate and blood circulation throughout the body; however, if your goal is to gain muscle mass, you'd do well to limit your cardio sessions. Limit each cardio session to 20 minute intervals while maintaining a low intensity throughout. This balance will provide all of the essential benefits cardiovascular activities have to offer without compromising muscle growth.

Don't Forget To Rest!

Making time for sleep is one of the most underrated factors in developing a healthy body composition or gaining muscle. It is easy to become anxious for gains that you try to do everything at once, leaving no time for friends, family, and most important... sleep!

Sleep is vital because during your sleep, muscle recovery is at its most efficient. Without adequate sleep, your body will break muscle down faster than it can repair. When you adopt a diet and exercise plan, consider adopting a resting plan as well. Make time for at least 7-8 hours of sleep each night where your body can properly recover from your workouts.

So, What Should Ectomorphs Do To Gain

Muscle?

For all of you busy ectomorphs who chose to skim this article and jump straight to the good stuff in the conclusion, here is a summary of the most important points all ectomorphs should remember:

• Understanding your body type first will allow you to set realistic and attainable goals.

• Food is your best friend. Eat plenty of carbs and protein, and don't neglect healthy fats. Aim to include at least one source of carbohydrates, proteins, and fats in every meal.

• If you're hitting the weights, focus on compound exercises that hit multiple muscle groups at once. Compound exercises build the most muscle mass and increase strength the fastest.

• You can include cardio into your exercise plan, but be careful not to overdo it. Limit your cardio sessions to 20 minutes intervals at a low intensity, and only a couple times per week.

• Remember that the more you exercise, the more you need to eat. Keep yourself in a caloric surplus while training heavy, and you'll see results.

• Get your 8 hours of sleep in every night. Your body already breaks itself down at a rapid pace. Sleep is what will help you repair muscle tissue and is crucial for muscle development.

It is important to understand that no matter which body type you have, you can achieve any fitness goal you set your mind to. The negative stigma associated with a certain body type only exists if we create it for ourselves. All body types will have its advantages and its disadvantages; what separates us is our will and our discipline to put forth the proper planning and positive mindset needed to succeed.

Ectomorph Diet Plan

So, here's your customized ectomorph diet plan to gain muscle. This diet plan for ectomorph is divided into six meals with three major meal and three minor meals or snacks.

Meal 1 – Breakfast

• 1 scoop whey isolate (I recommend MFF 100% Protein)

- 1 cup whole milk

- 1 large banana

- ¼ cup oats

- 2 tablespoon peanut butter

- Cocoa powder or chocolate syrup to taste

Blend all the above ingredients in a blender, and there you have it a calorie dense whey protein shake.

Nutrition Tip – If you ask me, I would recommend using MFF Whey Protein 100% because of its high protein content per scoop of serving. Besides, choose old-fashioned plain dry oats which are very easily available in the market these days. However, always keep in mind not to buy 'masala' or flavored oats for this type of protein shake. On top of these ingredients, you can even add a scoop of your favorite ice cream. Blending all the ingredients to a very fine size may take some time. Have patience.

Totals (Approximate)

• Calories – 630-660

• Protein – 40g

• Carbs – 60g

• Fat – 25g

Meal 2 – Snack

• 2 slices of whole wheat bread

• 2 tablespoon peanut butter

• 1 tablespoon jam

• 1 large banana

Nutrition Tip – Don't make a fool out of yourself by choosing white bread or multi-grain bread. Those are just processed garbage. Rather, use whole wheat bread whole grain bread. You can even replace banana with your favorite fruit of similar proportion.

Totals (Approximate)

- Calories – 500-530

- Protein – 15

- Carbs – 80-90

- Fats – 15

Meal 3 – Lunch

- 150 gram skinless chicken breast

- ½ cup brown rice

• ¼ cup green salad

• 1 tablespoon butter

Nutrition Tip – To cut down the fat content, I would suggest you purchase skinless chicken breast which is trimmed of fat. If you are buying chicken from a local chicken shop, you may ask the vendor to help you with that. Next up, opt for brown rice instead of white because of its low GI value. Don't forget to get your greens in this meal. A bowl of salad made with cabbage, beans, onions, cucumbers and carrots.

Totals (Approximate)

• Calories – 470-500

• Protein – 40g

• Carbs – 75g

• Fats – 6g

Meal 4 – Pre-Workout Shake

- 1 scoop whey protein

- 1 serving creatine monohydrate powder

- 1 cup fat-free milk

- 1 large banana

Nutrition Tip – The main purpose of this pre-workout shake is to channelize the flow of protein and other essential nutrients so as to create better blood flow to muscles and thereby long-lasting pump during the workout. Consume this shake 15-30 minutes before your workout begins.

Totals (Approximate)

- Calories – 350

• Protein – 26g

• Carbs – 60g

• Fat – 2g

Meal 5 – Post-Workout Shake

• 1 scoop whey protein

• 1 serving BCAA powder

• 1 scoop dextrose monohydrate

• 1 cup fat-free milk

• ¼ cup grapes

• 20 gram dark chocolate

Nutrition Tip – A post-workout shake is meant to revitalize and refuel the lost energy during the training session. While whey protein and bcaas are going to help you grow and recover, dextrose monohydrate aka fast carbs is going to replenish the lost glycogen stores during exercise. Moreover, fast carbs contain a good number of calories, a key necessity keeping in mind the diet for ectomorph.

Add your favorite fruit to the mix to get extra carbs. A surprise addition to the shake can be a medium piece of dark chocolate which is not only a powerful source of antioxidants but also helps in improving blood flow and soothing the mood.

Totals (Approximate)

• Calories – 560-600

• Protein – 27g

• Carbs – 100-120g

• Fats – 8g

Meal 6 – Dinner

• 150 gram skinless chicken breast

• Or similar proportion of tuna fish

• ½ cup brown rice

• ¼ cup green salad

• 1 tablespoon butter

Nutrition Tip – If you feel bored after eating chicken breast in the lunch, you can replace it with fish of a similar proportion. Needless to say, choose brown rice instead of the white one. One thing worth mentioning here is to try finishing your dinner by atleast 3-4 hours before bedtime. Since you are going to eat a considerable amount of carbs in the last meal of the day; it is not advisable to do it just before the sleep time. Even after dinner, go out for brisk walking. This little habit will not only burn calories but also help you recover faster.

Totals (Approximate)

- Calories – 450-480

- Protein – 40g

- Carbs – 60g

- Fat – 10g

Totals for an entire day of Ectomorph diet (Approximate)

- Calories – 3000-3100

- Protein – 160-180g

- Carbs – 400-450g

- Fat – 60-70g

Ectomorph Diet Recipes

Trying ectomorph diet-friendly recipes is a great way to explore new flavors and find new favorite dishes while looking after your health. In this part are nourishing ectomorph diet recipes for you to enjoy.

Hunter's Chicken

Prepartion time

1 hour 50 minutes

INGREDIENTS

- 8 skinless chicken thighs

- Sea salt and black pepper

- 8 bay leaves

- 3 sprigs fresh rosemary

- 3 cloves of garlic (1 crushed, 2 sliced)

- Half a bottle of chianti

- Olive oil

- 6 anchovy fillets

- Handful of green or black olives

- 2 x 400g tins of plum tomatoes

- Brown rice to serve

Instructions

1. Season the chicken with salt and pepper, add crushed garlic, rosemary, bay leaves and cover with the wine. Leave to marinate overnight or at least for an hour.

2. Preheat your oven to gas mark 4/180 degrees.

3. On the hob heat the sliced garlic until golden in a pan that is big enough for all the ingredients and can also go in the oven.

4. Add the anchovy's, olives, tomatoes (broken up), chicken thighs and the marinade.

5. Bring the mix to the boil and then remove from the heat, cover and place in the oven for 1.5 hours.

6. Skim off any oil that's collected on top and remove the rosemary sprigs and bay leaves.

7. Stir and enjoy! Serve with brown rice, salad or cannellini beans.

Dairy Free Carbonara

Prepartion time

25 minutes

INGREDIENTS

• 4 chicken breasts (chopped)

• 150g cashew nuts

• Paprika (to taste)

• 200g mushrooms (sliced)

• 100g pancetta (diced)

• Thyme (small bunch)

• 100ml white wine

• 400g dried spelt pasta

• 150ml hot water

• 400g broccoli

Instructions

1. Put the water on for your pasta.

2. Saute the pancetta with some thyme and black pepper for 3 minutes and then remove from the pan to a warm plate.

3. Add the chicken, salt, pepper and thyme to the same pan and saute for 4 minutes.

4. Remove the chicken to the warm plate with the pancetta.

5. Add the sliced mushrooms to the pan and saute for 3 minutes.

6. Mix the chicken and pancetta back in and add the white wine, cook for 5 to 7 minutes to reduce the wine.

7. Mix together the hot water, some seasoning, paprika and cashew nuts and blitz to a cream consistency, then add that to your pan and simmer gently.

8. Cook your pasta in your pan of hot water and, once cooked, mix with the chicken and pancetta.

9. Serve with 400g of steamed broccoli.

Flax Seed And Almond Bread

Prepartion time

45 minutes

INGREDIENTS

- 4 eggs

- 6 tbsp water

- 165g dark flax seeds

- 80g ground almonds

- 1 tsp baking powder

- 1 tsp salt

- 1 tsp caraway seeds

- 2 tsp honey

- 1/2 tsp xantham gum

- 2 tsp poppy seeds

- 35g sunflower seeds

- 35g black sesame seeds

• 20g flaked almonds

• 90g hazelnuts *

Instructions

1. Mix together the eggs and 3 tablespoons of water.

2. In a separate bowl mix together all the other ingredients with a further 3 tablespoons of water.

3. Then thoroughly mix your wet and dry ingredients before putting in a small loaf tin or tray and baking in the oven at 170 degrees for 30-40 minutes.

Fish And Chips With Avocado Dip

Prepartion time

50 minutes

INGREDIENTS

- 200g cod fillets

- 100g ⬚uinoa cooked & drained

- 50g spelt flour

- 3 eggs

- Handful of parsley chopped

- 10g black sesame seeds

116

- 200g sweet potato cut into wedges

- Sprig of rosemary

- 4 cloves of garlic, roughly chopped

- 2 tbsp rapeseed oil

- 1 ripe avocado

- Handful of coriander, chopped

- Juice of 1 lemon

- 1 tsp red pepper flakes

- Lemon wedges for garnish

Instructions

1. Pre-heat your oven to 200 degrees.

2. Mix the sweet potato wedges with the rapeseed oil, rosemary sprig, 2 of the garlic cloves and some seasoning.

3. Bake in the oven for 25-30 minutes until crispy.

4. Mix the quinoa, chopped parsley, sesame seeds and some seasoning in a bowl.

5. Whisk the eggs in another bowl.

6. Sieve the flour into another bowl.

7. First coat the cod in the flour, then the eggs and finish in the quinoa mix.

8. Bake in the oven for 12 minutes, or until cooked through.

9. While everything is cooking mix together the avocado, coriander, lemon juice, red pepper flakes and remaining 2 garlic cloves.

10. Blend together until you're happy with the consistency.

11. Serve the fish, chips and avocado dip finished with lemon wedges.

Chicken Pesto And Cashew

Prepartion time

20 minutes

INGREDIENTS

- 250g chicken, chopped

- 75g cashew nuts

- 150ml hot water

- 2 cloves garlic, crushed

- 200g courgettes, diced

- 120g cherry tomatoes

- 150g spinach

- 1 tbsp coconut oil

- 150g spelt pasta (or other pasta of your choice)

• Basil (to taste)

• 50g pine nuts

Instructions

1. Puree the cashew nuts with the hot water.

2. Put your pasta on to boil.

3. Saute the chicken gently for about 3 minutes in the coconut oil.

4. Add the garlic and cherry tomatoes and cook for 5 minutes.

5. Season and add the cashew nut mix and cook for a further 5 minutes.

6. Saute the courgettes in a separate pan so that they caramelise rather than stew.

7. Add the cooked courgettes, the spinach, pine nuts and basil 1 minute before the end.

8. Mix with the cooked pasta and serve.

Cajun Kebabs With Quinoa Salad

Prepartion time

30 minutes

INGREDIENTS

• 250g chicken pieces or large prawns

• 150g courgette, chopped into chunks

• 100g mushrooms, chopped into chunks

- 100g red pepper, chopped into chunks

- 100g cherry tomatoes

- 1 red onion, chopped into chunks

Cajun spice

- Sprig of thyme

- Sprig of rosemary

- 2 tsp garlic salt

- 1 tsp onion powder

- 2 1/2 tsp paprika

- 1 tsp cayenne pepper

- 1/2 tsp red pepper flakes

- 1 tsp black peppercorns

• 2 tbsp olive oil

Quinoa salad

• 100g quinoa

• 100g cucumber, finely diced

• Parsley to taste, chopped

• 1 lemon, juiced

Instructions

1. Preheat your oven to 180 degrees.

2. Chop the chicken and vegetables for the kebabs into large bite sized pieces (leave the prawns whole if you're using them instead of chicken).

3. Mix together all of the ingredients for the cajun spice and then use this to coat all the kebab vegetables and prawns or chicken.

4. Thread onto skewers in any order you like.

5. Bake the kebabs in the oven for 12 minutes, or until the chicken is cooked through.

6. Meanwhile, for the quinoa salad, cook your quinoa in a small pan (1 part quinoa to 2 parts cold water with a little salt) bring to the boil and simmer for around 10 minutes.

7. Drain and mix with the other salad ingredients.

Chicken Tikka

Prepartion time

30 minutes

INGREDIENTS

900g skinless chicken thighs

Spice mix

- 4g coriander seeds

- 15g cinnamon stick

- 2g fenugreek seeds

- 6g cumin seeds

- 6g peppercorns

- 1g cloves

- 2g nutmeg

- 2 bay leaves

- 5g turmeric

- 6g paprika

- 4g red pepper flakes

- 3 garlic cloves, pureed

- 15g ginger, pureed

- 2 lemons, juice only

- 100g coconut yoghurt

- Salt to taste

- Salad to serve

Instructions

1. Dry saute, grind and sieve the coriander seeds, cinnamon stick, fenugreek seeds, cumin seeds, peppercorns, cloves, nutmeg and bay leaves. If

127

you prefer to use already powdered versions, then add in smaller amounts of each.

2. To this mix, add the rest of the ingredients and then mix with the chicken thighs.

3. Leave to marinate for at least an hour, but ideally overnight.

4. Place on a wire rack with a baking tray underneath.

5. Bake at 180 degrees for 20-25 minutes, or until the chicken is cooked through (try not to overcook!).

6. Finish with a squeeze of lemon and serve with a salad.

Chicken Curry And Rice

Prepartion time

55 minutes

INGREDIENTS

• Spice mix

• 20g cinnamon stick

• 3g cardamon pods

• 4g peppercorns

• 1/2g coriander seeds

• 2g cumin seeds

- 2 bay leaves

- 3g turmeric

- 2g garam masala

- 3g paprika

- 200g onions, chopped or sliced

- 650g tomatoes, roughly chopped

- 180g red peppers, chopped

- 3 cloves of garlic (20g), pureed

- 20g ginger, pureed

- 650g skinless chicken thighs

- 30g tomato puree

- 200g brown basmati rice

- 1 lemon, wedges for garnish

• Small bunch of coriander, chopped

Instructions

1. Dry saute the cinnamon stick, cardamon pods, peppercorns, coriander seeds, cumin seeds and bay leaves for 4 minutes to release their oils and aroma.

2. Grind together and pass through a sieve. If you prefer to use ready powdered versions just use smaller amounts of each.

3. Add the turmeric, garam masala and paprika.

4. Put to one side. Saute the onions gently for about 10 minutes until they're nicely browned.

5. Add the peppers and saute gently for a further 4 minutes.

6. Add the garlic and ginger purees and cook for 2 minutes.

7. Add the chopped tomatoes and gently simmer for 30-40 minutes.

8. Let it break down into a sauce.

9. Meanwhile cook the brown rice according to the packet instructions.

10. Once the tomatoes have broken down add the chicken and spice mix.

11. Cook for a further 15 minutes (or until the chicken is cooked through, keep it nice and moist).

12. Serve with the brown rice and finish with a generous handful of chopped coriander and squeeze of lemon. You could add a little natural yoghurt or coconut milk if you like.

Spiced Chicken On Quinoa

Prepartion time

1 hour 40 minutes

INGREDIENTS

• 800g chicken breasts, each cut into 3

• Marinade

• 4 tbsp lemon juice

• 4 cloves of garlic, crushed

• 20g ginger, crushed

• 1 tsp turmeric

• 1 tsp paprika

• 1 tsp cumin

• 1 tsp sumac

• 1tsp ground cardamon

133

- 1 onion, sliced

- 2 red peppers, sliced

- 200g raw quinoa

Sprig of thyme

- 400ml hot chicken stock

- 600g tender stem broccoli to serve

- Warm aubergine salad

- 1 aubergine (cut & salt 20 mins before)

- 6 tomatoes, chopped

- 1 tsp nutmeg

- 2 tsp lemon juice

Instructions

1. Mix the chicken and marinade ingredients and leave for at least an hour, but ideally overnight. If

marinading for an hour, at the same time chop and salt the aubergine for the salad. Remember to rinse the aubergine before using.

2. To make the main dish you need a pan or dish that is large enough to hold all the ingredients and can go in the oven. Cover the bottom of the dish with raw ⬚uinoa.

3. Then add the onions and peppers. Add the thyme and a little salt and pepper.

4. Arrange the marinaded chicken over the top.

5. Finally, pour over the hot stock until the chicken is half covered.

6. Bake for 45 minutes at 180 degrees. Meanwhile, to make the aubergine salad, saute the aubergine for 20 minutes, then add some black pepper, the tomatoes, nutmeg and lemon.

7. Add a little water, bring to the boil and simmer for 25 minutes.

8. Serve with the steamed broccoli.

Mexican Casserole With Sweet Potato

Prepartion time

1 hour

INGREDIENTS

• 100g chorizo, chopped into small cubes

• 600g skinless chicken thighs deboned

• 150g onions, roughly chopped

• 100g red pepper, sliced

• 100g green pepper, sliced

- 4 garlic cloves, finely chopped

- 200ml red wine

- 400g tomatoes, roughly chopped

- 3 tsp tomato puree

- 80g black olives

- 2 tsp paprika

- 2 tsp cayenne pepper

- 1 tsp ground cinnamon

- 2tsp red pepper flakes

- 200ml chicken stock

- 400g sweet potato, washed and sliced

- Sprig of oregano

- 1 tsp garlic salt

• Pinch crushed black pepper

• 2 tbsp rapeseed oil

• Lime, cut into wedges for garnish

Instructions

1. Salute the chicken and chorizo for 6 minutes until well sealed.

2. Remove from the pan and pop to one side.

3. In the same pan gently saute the onions and peppers for 10 minutes.

4. Add the garlic and cook for a further 2 minutes.

5. Add the red wine, bring to the boil and reduce so it becomes sticky.

6. Add the tomatoes and tomato puree.

7. Add all the spices and some seasoning and cook for a further 3 minutes.

8. Add the stock, bring to the boil and simmer for 15 minutes.

9. Mix the sliced sweet potatoes with the oregano, garlic salt, black pepper and rapeseed oil.

10. Add the chicken and chorizo back in and pour the entire mix into a casserole dish.

11. Arrange the sliced potato over the top.

12. Bake in the oven at 180 degrees for 20-30 minutes, until the potatoes are crispy and cooked through.

13. Serve with some freshly squeezed lime.

Classic Bolognese

Prepartion time

50 minutes

INGREDIENTS

- 500g beef or pork mince

- 1 large onion

- 1 green pepper

- 2 courgettes

- 4-5 cloves of garlic

- Coconut oil

- 200g mushrooms

- 700g jar of passata

- 2 tbsp tomato puree

- 300g spelt or wholegrain pasta

Instructions

1. Saute the mince in a little coconut oil and drain in a colander and place to one side.

2. Saute all the vegetables and then add the mince back to the pan and add the passata and tomato puree.

3. Simmer for 30-45 minutes before serving with your choice of wholegrain pasta.

Chicken Tray Bake

Prepartion time

50 minutes

INGREDIENTS

- 6 boneless, skinless chicken thighs

- 1 red pepper, roughly chopped

- 5 cloves of garlic, roughly chopped

- 1 courgette, chopped into large chunks

- 1 red onion, roughly chopped

- 1 tbsp rapeseed oil

- 15 cherry tomatoes, left whole

- Third of a block of feta, cubed

- 3-4 handfuls of spinach

- 400g tin of beans of your choice (mixed, haricot, kidney, borlotti etc)

- Salt and pepper

- Handful of fresh thyme

- 2 tsp smoked paprika

• Drizzle of balsamic vinegar

Instructions

1. Preheat the oven to 180 degrees. Put the chicken, red pepper, garlic, courgette, red onion and tomatoes in an oven proof tray and drizzle with the rapeseed oil.

2. Season with the smoked paprika, thyme, salt and pepper.

3. Place in the oven for 25 minutes.

4. Take out the tray and add the tin of beans and put back in the oven for 10 minutes.

5. Then increase the oven temperature to 200 degrees and cook for a further 5 minutes.

6. Take out of the oven and add the feta, spinach and drizzle of balsamic vinegar, mix well so that the feta starts to melt and the spinach wilts.

Banana, Chocolate & Nut Bread

Prepartion time

1 hour 10 minutes

INGREDIENTS

- 60g Coconut flour

- 100g Dark chocolate

- 25g Almonds

- 20g Sunflower seeds

- 1.5 tsp Baking powder

- 1 tsp Vanilla essence

• 4 Large ripe Bananas

• 4 Medium eggs

• 3 tbsp Coconut oil

Instructions

1. Heat the oven to 180 degrees.

2. Mix together the coconut flour, dark chocolate, almonds, sunflower seeds and baking powder in a mixer.

3. Then add the vanilla essence, bananas (reserve a few slices to decorate the top), eggs and coconut oil and mix again.

4. Once mixed, pour into a lined loaf tin, top with the reserved slices of banana and bake in the oven for 50 to 60 minutes (or until a cake skewer or knife comes out clean).

5. Cool on a rack before turning out of the tin.

Potato Salad With Anchovy & Quails Egg

Prepartion time

15 minutes

INGREDIENTS

• 4 Quails eggs

• 100g green beans

• 100g new potatoes, halved or quartered

• 1 anchovy, finely chopped

• 1 tbsp chopped parsley

• 1 tbsp chopped chives

• Juice of half a lemon

Instructions

1. Put the potatoes in a pan of cold water, bring to the boil and simmer until the potatoes are cooked.

2. Once ready, drain in a colander and leave to cool.

3. Meanwhile, bring a medium pan of water to a simmer.

4. Lower the 🔲uail eggs into the water and cook for 2 minutes.

5. Lift the 🔲uail eggs out with a slotted spoon and place into cold water.

6. Add the beans to the pan you used for the eggs and simmer for 4 minutes until tender.

7. Remove from the pan with a slotted spoon and plunge into cold water with the eggs.

147

8. Once the potatoes are ready, peel the eggs and cut them in half.

9. Then, toss the potatoes and beans with the chopped anchovies, herbs, and lemon juice.

10. Then top with the peeled quail eggs and serve.

Immune Boosting Smoothie

Prepartion time

5 minutes

INGREDIENTS

• 50g Apricots

• Half an Avocado

• 20g Almonds

• 50g Berries

• Handful of Kale

• 20g Brazil nuts

• 30g Watermelon

• 20g Walnuts

• 10g Pumpkin seeds

• 40g Banana

• Coconut water

Instructions

1. Add all of the ingredients to your mixer, top up with coconut water and blend.

Heart Health Smoothie

Prepartion time

5 minutes

INGREDIENTS

• 100g Berries

• Handful of Kale

• Handful of Spinach

• 20g Almonds

- 10g Sesame seeds

- 30g Oat bran

- 10g Pumpkin seeds

- Half an avocado

- 20g Cucumber

- 20g Apricots

- 20g Nuts

- Probiotic (as pre label)

- 20g Blackcurrants

- 20g Strawberries

Instructions

1. Add all of the ingredients to your mixer, top up with coconut water and blend.

Detox Smoothie

Prepartion time

5 minutes

INGREDIENTS

- 50g Beetroot

- 50g Celery

- 50g Apple

- Handful of Spinach

- Spirulina (as per label)

- Chlorella (as per label)

- 30g Carrots

- 40g Citrus fruits

- Cold green tea

Instructions

1. Add all of the ingredients to your mixer, top up with cold green tea and blend.

Anti-Ageing Smoothie

Prepartion time

5 minutes

INGREDIENTS

• 20g Cashew nuts

• 10g Sesame seeds

• 10g Sunflower seeds

• 50g Oats

• 20g Pumpkins seeds

• Big handful of Spinach

- 20g Brazil nuts

- 50g Citrus fruits

- Half an Avocado

- Coconut water

Instructions

1. Add all of the ingredients to your mixer, top up with coconut water and blend.

Skin Smoothie

Prepartion time

5 minutes

INGREDIENTS

- 40g Red apple

- 40g Berries

- 15g Almonds

- 15g Cashews

- Handful of Swiss chard

- 20g Brazil nuts

- 20g Goji berries

- Coconut water

Instructions

1. Add all of the ingredients to your mixer, top up with coconut water and blend.

Brain Boosting Smoothie

Prepartion time

5 minutes

INGREDIENTS

- 20g Sunflower seeds

- Handful of Spinach

- 50g Cantaloupe melon

- Handful of Kale

- 20g Almonds

- 20g Flax seeds

- Half an Avocado

- Coconut water

Instructions

1. Add all of the ingredients to your mixer, top up with coconut water and blend.

Bone Strengthen Smoothie

Prepartion time

5 minutes

INGREDIENTS

• Small handful of Spinach

• Small handful of Kale

• Small handful of Collard Greens

• 20g Wheatbran

• 20g Almonds

• 20g Cashews

• 40g Papaya

• Handful of Swiss Chard

• Coconut water

Instructions

1. Add all of the ingredients to your mixer, top up
with coconut water and blend.

Sleep Well Smoothie

Prepartion time

5 minutes

INGREDIENTS

20g Dates

20g Cashews

30g Oats

Spirulina (as per label)

15g Pumpkin seeds

Handful of Swiss chard

Handful of Spinach

Handful of Collard greens

1 tsp Cinnamon

Almond milk

Instructions

1. Add all of the ingredients to your mixer, top up with almond milk and blend.

Stress Busting Smoothie

Prepartion time

5 minutes

INGREDIENTS

• 20g Nuts

• 10g Seeds

• Handful of Spinach

• Half an Avocado

• 50g Yoghurt

• 30g Cucumber

- 20g Blackcurrants

- 20g Strawberries

- Coconut water

Instructions

1. Add all of the ingredients to your blender, top up with coconut water and blend.

Energy Boosting Smoothie

Prepartion time

5 minutes

INGREDIENTS

- 20g Nuts

- 10g Sunflower seeds

- Handful of spinach

- 100ml Grape juice

- Half an Avocado

- 50g Cantaloupe melon

- 30g Blackcurrants

- Handful of Swiss chard

Instructions

1. Add all of the ingredients to your mixer and blend.

Sweet Cinnamon Balls

Prepartion time

15 minutes

INGREDIENTS

- 120g Mixed nuts (we used Brazil nuts, walnuts & hazelnuts)

- 45g dried cranberries

- 120g pitted dates

- Zest of 1 lime & a little juice

- 20g Sunflower seeds

- 1 tbsp Cinnamon

Instructions

1. Pulse the nuts in a mixer until chopped.

2. Then add the dried cranberries and pitted dates and mix further until starting to bind together.

3. Add the lime zest and a little of the juice and process until sticky.

162

4. Take pieces of the mixture and roll into balls.

5. Add sunflower seeds to the now empty mixer and pulse until fine, then add the cinnamon.

6. Coat the balls in the mix of sunflower seeds and cinnamon.

7. Store in the fridge, will keep for up to 2 weeks.

Chicken With Mushrooms

Prepartion time

25 minutes

INGREDIENTS

• Rapeseed oil

• 500g boneless skinless chicken thighs (kept whole)

- 1 tbsp flour

- 50g cubed pancetta

- 300g button mushrooms, halved

- 2 large shallots chopped

- 250ml chicken stock

- 1 tbsp white wine vinegar

- 50g frozen peas

- Handful chopped parsley

- Green vegetables to serve

Instructions

1. Heat 1 tablespoon of oil in a large frying pan, dust the chicken with the flour and add to the pan.

2. Once brown on all sides, remove from the pan and place to one side.

3. Add the pancetta and mushrooms to the same pan and cook until soft, then remove to rest with the chicken.

4. Add a teaspoon of oil to the same pan with the shallots and cook for a minute or so.

5. Then add the stock and vinegar.

6. Bring to the boil for a couple of minutes before adding the chicken, pancetta and mushrooms.

7. Simmer for 15 minutes.

8. Finally, add the frozen peas and cook for about 2 minutes before adding the chopped parsley to finish.

9. Serve with green vegetables.

Chicken Kebab With Quinoa Salad

Prepartion time

20 minutes

INGREDIENTS

For the kebabs:

- 2 kebabs per person

- 2 Chicken breasts cut into bite sized pieces

- 1 Red pepper, cut into pieces to skewer

- 1 Courgette, sliced

- Handful of Cherry tomatoes

- 2 Garlic cloves, finely chopped

- 1 tbsp Fresh Thyme, finely chopped

For the salad:

• Cherry tomatoes

• Cucumber

• Red Pepper

• Feta

• Black olives

• Small avocado

• 2 small cloves of garlic, finely chopped

• Fresh red chilli, de-seeded and finely chopped

• Handful of fresh Coriander, chopped

• Juice of 1 lemon

• Cooked Quinoa

• 2 tbsp Olive oil

Instructions

1. Soak your kebab sticks in water to prevent them burning then make your kebabs by adding chicken, red pepper, courgette slices and whole cherry tomatoes.

2. Marinade the kebabs with garlic, thyme and lemon then bake in the oven at 180 for 12 to 15 minutes.

3. To make the salad, finely chop all of the ingredients. You want everything to be a similar size, except for the chilli and garlic, which will be more finely chopped.

4. Mix the salad ingredients with your Quinoa, some olive oil and salt and pepper.

Beef Bourguignon With Quinoa

Prepartion time

15 minutes

INGREDIENTS

- 300g Sirloin steak, sliced into strips

- 150g Chantenay carrots

- 1 x Onion, diced

- 1 tbsp Fresh thyme, finely chopped

- 150ml Red wine

- 150ml Beef stock

- 1 tbsp Tomato puree

- 1 x Courgette, chopped to a similar size as the carrots

• 100g Quinoa

Instructions

1. In a large frying pan lightly sauté the sirloin steak (keep it pink) and then place to one side.

2. Steam the carrots. In the same pan you used for the steak, sauté the onions with some thyme.

3. Add the red wine and simmer to reduce.

4. Add beef stock and tomato puree.

5. Again, simmer to reduce.

6. Add chopped courgettes to the pan of steaming carrots for the last 4 minutes.

7. In a separate pan cook your quinoa.

8. Add the steak back into the pan and mix well.

9. Serve with the quinoa and steamed vegetables.

Sauted Potatoes With Avocado & Eggs

Prepartion time

15 minutes

INGREDIENTS

• Handful of new potatoes, sliced

• 1 tbsp Coconut oil

• 100g Cherry tomatoes, halved

• Small avocado

• Lemon juice

• 3 x Large eggs

Instructions

1. In a large frying pan sauté the new potatoes in the coconut oil until they're cooked through, golden and crispy.

171

2. Meanwhile, in a separate pan cook the cherry tomatoes.

3. Mash an avocado with some seasoning and a little lemon juice.

4. Gently scramble your eggs (without any milk or butter).

5. Serve in a stack with potatoes, avocado, cooked tomatoes and finished with your scrambled eggs.

Cod On Aubergine & Tomato Pulp

Prepartion time

20 minutes

INGREDIENTS

- 1 x Onion, finely chopped

- 150g Cherry tomatoes, halved

- 50g Black olives, sliced

- 1 x Aubergine, cut into thick slices

- 2 x Cod fillets

- 200g Spinach

- Dressing of olive oil, lemon juice & seasoning

Instructions

1. Sauté the onion in a large frying pan until soft and transluscent, add the cherry tomatoes and cook for a couple more minutes and then add the black olives.

2. Keep warm on a low heat.

173

3. In a separate pan, sauté the sliced aubergines to add a bit of colour and then place to one side.

4. Next sauté the seasoned cod fillets with a little bit of thyme for a minute or two on each side and then place the cod and aubergine slices in the oven and bake until the cod is cooked through (about 15 minutes, depending on the size of your fillets).

5. When the fish is nearly ready, gently steam the spinach.

6. To serve, place the aubergine slices on a warmed plate, top with the wilted spinach, the tomato and olive mix, followed by the cod fillet finished with a little of your dressing (mixed to a 2:1 ratio).

Mildly Spiced Chicken & Rice

174

Prepartion time

20 minutes

INGREDIENTS

• 1 Onion, finely chopped

• 2 Cloves of garlic, finely chopped

• 1 Red pepper, sliced

• 6 x Chicken thighs (skinless and boneless) cut into large pieces

• 2 tsp of curry or chilli powder

• 100g White rice

• 150g Cherry tomatoes, halved

• 500ml Chicken stock

• 100g Spinach

Instructions

175

1. Saute the onion and garlic in a large frying pan for a couple of minutes and then add the red pepper, chicken thighs, the spices and some seasoning, the raw white rice, cherry tomatoes and chicken stock (enough to cover the rice).

2. Bring to the boil and simmer for about 15 minutes until the chicken and rice are cooked through.

3. Just before you take off the heat add the spinach for 1 minute, so it wilts nicely in the heat.

Spicy Chicken & Brown Rice

Prepartion time

1 hour

INGREDIENTS

• 8 Chicken thighs (remove skin & bone, but keep whole)

• 1 Onion, finely sliced

• 1 tsp Cayenne pepper

• 1 tsp Sweet paprika

• 1 tsp Cumin

• 1 tsp Garam masala

• 1 tsp Cinnamon

• 1 tsp Turmeric

• 200g Brown rice

• 200g Cherry tomatoes, halved

• 400g Chick peas

• 500-750ml Hot chicken stock

- 100g Spinach

- Coriander to garnish

Instructions

1. Skin and de-bone your chicken thighs, if not already done. Finely slice the onions.

2. Measure and mix the spices before coating the chicken thighs with them. In a large saucepan that can go in the oven add the brown rice, the onion and garlic, chicken thighs, cherry tomatoes and hot chicken stock (you need enough stock to cover the rice and sit halfway up the chicken).

3. Place the lid on top and place in the oven at 180 degrees until cooked through (45 min to an hour).

4. Add the spinach right at the end and allow it to gently steam in the heat with the lid on.

5. Garnish with coriander & enjoy!

Avocado On Toast With Poached Eggs

Prepartion time

15 minutes

INGREDIENTS

• 2 x small pieces of pumpernickel or rye bread

• Half a mashed avocado

• Handful of cherry tomatoes

• 2 x Large eggs

Instructions

1. Lightly toast two small pieces of pumpernickel or rye bread (if you can't get either of these then stoneground wholemeal bread is best).

2. Lightly saute your cherry tomatoes and mash half an avocado with some seasoning and a little bit of lemon juice.

3. Top one piece of toast with the cherry tomatoes, the other with the avocado and finish each with a softly poached egg.